DEFY CANCER

NAVIGATING DIAGNOSIS, TREATMENT, AND RECOVERY WITH CONFIDENCE

SAMUEL EKPENYONG

ISBN: 9798334178380

samuelekpenyong.mkd@gmail.com

www.amazon.com/author/samek-books

Forward

It is with great pleasure that I introduce this comprehensive guide on cancer prevention and management. Cancer continues to be one of the most pressing health challenges of our time, affecting millions worldwide and demanding a multifaceted approach to mitigate its impact.

This book represents a meticulous exploration into the intricacies of cancer prevention and management, offering a structured framework to understand the complexities of this disease. From its fundamental definitions to the latest advancements in treatment modalities, each chapter is meticulously crafted to provide both healthcare professionals and the general public with invaluable insights and actionable knowledge.

The chapters traverse through critical topics such as the causes and risk factors contributing to cancer, the significance of early detection and screening, and the pivotal role of lifestyle modifications including diet, exercise, and smoking cessation. Moreover, it delves into emerging areas of cancer prevention, such as immunization against specific cancers and the influence of environmental and occupational exposures.

Importantly, this book doesn't merely address the physical aspects of cancer but also underscores the psychological and social dimensions, recognizing the profound impact on patients' lives and emphasizing supportive strategies and survivorship care.

As a scientist and practitioner in the field, I commend the authors for their dedication in compiling this essential resource. It serves not only as a guide for healthcare providers navigating the complexities of cancer care, but also as a beacon of hope and knowledge for individuals seeking to understand and proactively manage their health.

I trust that this book will inspire readers to engage actively in cancer prevention efforts, foster informed discussions among healthcare professionals, and ultimately contribute to the collective endeavor of reducing the global burden of cancer.

Dr. Michael Jakes Ph.D.

University of Uyo Teaching Hospital,

Akwa Ibom State, Nigeria.

Table of Contents

CHAPTER ONE

Introduction

Cancer, a pervasive and intricate constellation of diseases, stands as one of the foremost challenges to global health in the modern era. Defined by the unregulated growth and spread of abnormal cells, cancer disrupts the delicate balance of cellular processes essential for normal tissue function. This disruption leads to the formation of malignant tumors and can result in systemic effects that profoundly impact an individual's health and well-being.

The diversity of cancer types reflects the complex interplay of genetic, environmental, and lifestyle factors that contribute to its development. From the cellular level to clinical manifestations, understanding the biology of cancer requires a nuanced appreciation of its heterogeneous nature. This complexity underscores the necessity of tailored approaches to diagnosis, treatment, and prevention.

Moreover, cancer's global footprint is undeniable. It transcends geographical boundaries, affecting populations across continents and demographics. Its prevalence continues to rise, fueled by demographic shifts, industrialization, and changing patterns of behavior. As societies age and lifestyles evolve, the burden of cancer grows, placing significant strains on healthcare systems worldwide.

In this context, the exploration of cancer encompasses not only scientific and clinical dimensions but also socio-economic and public health perspectives. It demands comprehensive strategies that integrate advancements in research with efforts in prevention, early detection, and access to quality care. By elucidating the fundamental aspects of cancer biology, epidemiology, and impact, this chapter seeks to provide a robust foundation for understanding the ongoing challenges and opportunities in the fight against cancer.

Through concerted global efforts in research, education, and policy, the quest to conquer cancer remains a compelling imperative, driven by the shared goal of alleviating suffering and improving outcomes for individuals and communities affected by this formidable disease.

Definition of Cancer

Cancer is a complex and multifaceted disease characterized by the uncontrolled growth and spread of abnormal cells within the body. According to renowned scholars in oncology, such as Douglas Hanahan and

Robert A. Weinberg, cancer originates from genetic mutations that disrupt the regulatory mechanisms governing cell division and growth. These mutations enable cells to evade normal cellular checkpoints that would otherwise trigger apoptosis (programmed cell death) in damaged or abnormal cells.

Fundamentally, cancerous cells exhibit traits such as sustained proliferative signaling, insensitivity to growth inhibitors, evasion of apoptosis, limitless replicative potential, sustained angiogenesis (formation of new blood vessels), and tissue invasion and metastasis. These hallmarks, as described by Hanahan and Weinberg in their seminal paper, highlight the biological complexities underlying cancer development and progression.

Moreover, the heterogeneity of cancer types reflects the diverse tissues and organs from which tumors can arise. Carcinomas, originating from epithelial tissues, represent the most common form of cancer, accounting for approximately 80-90% of cases. Other types include sarcomas (arising from connective tissues), lymphomas (involving lymphatic tissues), and leukemias (originating in blood-forming tissues).

From a clinical perspective, cancer presents significant challenges in diagnosis, treatment, and management. Early detection plays a critical role in improving outcomes, as timely intervention can mitigate the disease's progression and enhance survival rates. Diagnostic modalities range from imaging techniques such as computed tomography (CT) and magnetic resonance imaging (MRI) to molecular diagnostics that analyze genetic and biochemical markers indicative of cancerous growth.

In summary, the definition of cancer

encompasses not only its molecular and cellular underpinnings but also its profound impact on individual health and global public health. By integrating insights from leading scholars and clinicians, this chapter aims to provide a comprehensive framework for understanding the complexities of cancer biology, its clinical manifestations, and the ongoing efforts to advance treatments and improve patient outcomes.

Types of cancers

1. Carcinomas:

- Carcinomas are cancers that arise from epithelial cells, which are cells that line the surfaces and cavities of organs throughout the body. They are the most common type of cancer and can occur in various organs, including the skin, lungs, breasts, prostate, and colon.

2. **Sarcomas:**

- Sarcomas develop from mesenchymal cells, which are found in connective tissues such as bones, muscles, cartilage, and fat. These cancers are less common than carcinomas and can be further categorized into types like osteosarcoma (bone cancer) and leiomyosarcoma (smooth muscle cancer).

3. **Lymphomas:**

- Lymphomas are cancers that originate in the lymphatic system, which is part of the body's immune system. They typically begin in lymphocytes (white blood cells) and can affect lymph nodes, bone marrow, spleen, and other lymphatic tissues. Hodgkin lymphoma and non-Hodgkin lymphoma are the two main types.

4. **Leukemias:**

- Leukemias are cancers that begin in blood-forming tissues, such as the bone marrow, and result in large numbers of abnormal blood cells being produced and entering the bloodstream. They can be categorized as acute (rapidly progressing) or chronic (slowly progressing), and types include acute myeloid leukemia (AML), chronic lymphocytic leukemia (CLL), and others.

5. Central Nervous System (CNS) Cancers:

   - These cancers occur in the brain and spinal cord and can be primary (originating in the CNS) or secondary (metastasizing from other parts of the body). Gliomas, meningiomas, and medulloblastomas are examples of CNS cancers.

6. Gastrointestinal Cancers:

   - This category includes cancers of the gastrointestinal tract, such as the esophagus, stomach, liver, pancreas, gallbladder, colon, and rectum. Each type of gastrointestinal cancer has unique risk factors, symptoms, and treatment approaches.

7. Genitourinary Cancers:

- Genitourinary cancers affect the urinary tract (bladder, kidneys, ureters) and reproductive organs (prostate, testes, ovaries). Examples include bladder cancer, kidney cancer, prostate cancer, and ovarian cancer.

8. Endocrine Cancers:

- These cancers originate in endocrine glands, which produce hormones that regulate various bodily functions. Examples include thyroid cancer, adrenal cancer, and pancreatic neuroendocrine tumors.

9. Respiratory Cancers:

- Respiratory cancers primarily affect the lungs and respiratory system. Lung cancer is the most common type, but other types include cancers of the trachea, bronchi, and pleura (lining of the lungs).

10. **Skin Cancers:**

   - Skin cancers develop from skin cells and are mainly caused by exposure to ultraviolet (UV) radiation from sunlight or tanning beds. The most common types are basal cell carcinoma, squamous cell carcinoma, and melanoma.

Each type of cancer has distinct characteristics, behaviors, risk factors, and treatment options. Understanding these differences is crucial for accurate diagnosis, effective treatment planning, and improving outcomes for patients affected by cancer.

Global Impact and Prevalence of Cancer

Cancer represents a significant global health challenge, exerting a profound impact on individuals, communities, and healthcare systems worldwide. Understanding its prevalence and distribution is essential for effective prevention, early detection, treatment, and resource allocation.

Prevalence and Incidence

The prevalence of cancer continues to rise globally, driven by factors such as aging populations, lifestyle changes, and environmental exposures. According to the World Health Organization (WHO), cancer is one of the leading causes of morbidity and mortality worldwide, accounting for an estimated 10 million deaths annually.

Incidence rates vary significantly across regions and countries, influenced by demographic trends, socio-economic development, healthcare infrastructure, and access to screening and treatment services. High-income countries generally report higher incidence rates due to better diagnostic capabilities and longer life expectancy, whereas low- and middle-income countries face rising burdens as they undergo epidemiological transitions and adopt Western lifestyles.

Global Distribution

Certain types of cancer exhibit geographical variations in incidence and mortality rates. For example, lung cancer is more prevalent in countries with high smoking rates, while liver cancer is disproportionately common in regions where chronic hepatitis B and C infections are prevalent. Breast cancer rates vary due to factors such as reproductive behaviors, access to mammography screening, and genetic predispositions.

Impact on Health Systems

The economic burden of cancer is substantial, encompassing direct healthcare costs (diagnosis, treatment, and supportive care), indirect costs (lost productivity), and intangible costs (pain and suffering). This burden strains healthcare budgets and necessitates prioritization of cancer prevention and control efforts.

Challenges and Opportunities

Addressing the global impact of cancer requires comprehensive strategies that integrate prevention, early detection, diagnosis, treatment, palliative care, and survivorship support. Key challenges include disparities in access to healthcare services, limited resources in low-resource settings, and barriers to implementing evidence-based interventions.

Despite these challenges, advances in

cancer research, technology, and public health initiatives offer opportunities for progress. Innovations in precision medicine, immunotherapy, and targeted therapies hold promise for improving treatment outcomes and quality of life for cancer patients worldwide.

Conclusion

In summary, cancer's global impact underscores the urgent need for coordinated action at local, national, and international levels. By enhancing cancer surveillance, strengthening healthcare systems, promoting healthy lifestyles, and expanding access to essential medicines and technologies, the global community can mitigate the burden of cancer and improve outcomes for millions of individuals affected by this complex disease.

CHAPTER TWO

Causes and Risk Factors

Understanding the intricate web of factors contributing to disease onset is paramount in the study of health sciences. This chapter delves into the multifaceted elements influencing the development of various conditions, with a particular focus on genetic predisposition, lifestyle factors, and environmental influences.

GENETIC PREDISPOSITION

Genetic predisposition constitutes a pivotal aspect of disease etiology, intertwining inherited traits with the susceptibility to various health conditions. At its core, genetic predisposition encompasses the presence of specific genetic variations or mutations that can heighten an individual's likelihood of developing certain diseases. These genetic factors may act independently or synergistically with environmental influences, shaping disease onset and progression.

The study of genetic predisposition delves into the intricate mechanisms by which genetic variations influence disease susceptibility. Advances in genomic research have unveiled a spectrum of genetic markers, ranging from single nucleotide polymorphisms (SNPs) to complex gene-environment interactions. These insights illuminate the genetic architecture underlying diseases such as cancer, cardiovascular disorders, neurodegenerative conditions, and autoimmune diseases.

Importantly, genetic predisposition does not solely determine disease manifestation but rather interacts dynamically with environmental factors and lifestyle choices.

This interaction underscores the concept of "genetic susceptibility," where genetic predisposition amplifies the impact of environmental exposures, lifestyle habits, and other external influences on disease risk.

Furthermore, genetic predisposition underscores the importance of personalized medicine and precision healthcare approaches. By identifying individuals at heightened genetic risk, healthcare providers can tailor screening programs, preventive measures, and therapeutic interventions to mitigate risks and optimize health outcomes. This paradigm shift from a one-size-fits-all approach to personalized medicine holds promise for improving diagnostic accuracy, treatment efficacy, and patient-centered care.

In conclusion, genetic predisposition represents a foundational pillar in understanding disease causation and individualized health management. As genomic technologies continue to evolve, unraveling the complexities of genetic predisposition will pave the way for targeted interventions that promote health resilience and disease prevention across diverse populations.

LIFESTYLE FACTORS

Lifestyle factors exert profound influence on health outcomes, encompassing a broad spectrum of daily habits and behaviors that significantly impact disease risk and overall well-being. Central to this concept are dietary patterns, physical activity levels, sleep hygiene, and substance use, each playing distinct roles in shaping individual health trajectories.

Dietary habits constitute a cornerstone of lifestyle factors, with nutritional choices profoundly influencing metabolic health, immune function, and disease susceptibility. A diet rich in fruits, vegetables, whole grains, and lean proteins provides essential nutrients and antioxidants that bolster cellular resilience and mitigate chronic diseases such as cardiovascular disorders, diabetes, and certain cancers. Conversely, diets high in processed foods, saturated fats, and added sugars contribute to metabolic dysregulation, inflammation, and increased risk of obesity-related conditions.

Physical activity stands as another critical determinant of health, exerting multifaceted benefits across physiological and psychological domains. Regular exercise promotes cardiovascular fitness, enhances musculoskeletal strength, and optimizes metabolic processes, thereby reducing the incidence of cardiovascular disease, osteoporosis, and type 2 diabetes. Moreover, physical activity fosters neuroplasticity and mental well-being, mitigating stress, anxiety, and depression while promoting cognitive function and overall quality of life.

Adequate sleep hygiene constitutes an often-overlooked yet crucial aspect of healthy living. Quality sleep supports immune function, facilitates tissue repair, and regulates hormone production, influencing metabolic processes and cognitive performance. Chronic sleep deprivation, conversely, disrupts these physiological rhythms, predisposing individuals to obesity, cardiovascular disease, mood disorders, and impaired immune responses.

Furthermore, lifestyle factors encompass behaviors such as tobacco and alcohol consumption, which exert significant health ramifications. Cigarette smoking remains a leading preventable cause of death worldwide, contributing to lung cancer, respiratory diseases, and cardiovascular disorders. Similarly, excessive alcohol consumption correlates with liver disease, hypertension, and increased cancer risks, underscoring the importance of moderation or abstinence in maintaining optimal health.

In sum, lifestyle factors collectively constitute modifiable determinants of health that empower individuals to proactively enhance their well-being and reduce disease burden. By promoting balanced dietary choices, regular physical activity, adequate sleep, and avoidance of harmful substances, healthcare practitioners and policymakers alike can foster a culture of preventive healthcare, ultimately improving population health outcomes and reducing healthcare costs.

ENVIRONMENTAL FACTORS

Environmental factors encompass a broad array of external influences that significantly impact human health, ranging from air and water quality to occupational hazards and climate change. These factors play a pivotal role in shaping disease patterns and public health outcomes, highlighting the interconnectedness between human health and environmental sustainability.

Air quality stands as a critical environmental determinant of health, with exposure to pollutants such as particulate matter, nitrogen dioxide, and ozone contributing to respiratory ailments, cardiovascular diseases, and exacerbating conditions like asthma. Urbanization, industrial activities, and vehicular emissions further underscore the importance of regulatory measures and technological advancements aimed at reducing air pollution levels and safeguarding respiratory health.

Water quality represents another vital facet of environmental health, with access to clean water and sanitation facilities serving as fundamental prerequisites for disease prevention and community well-being. Contamination from pathogens, heavy metals, and chemical pollutants poses significant public health risks, contributing to waterborne diseases such as cholera, dysentery, and hepatitis. Efforts to improve water infrastructure, implement water treatment technologies, and promote safe hygiene practices are crucial in ensuring equitable access to clean water and reducing global disease burdens.

Additionally, occupational hazards present distinct challenges to worker health and safety, encompassing exposures to hazardous chemicals, biological agents, ergonomic stressors, and physical hazards in various workplace settings. Occupational diseases, injuries, and long-term health impacts underscore the importance of workplace safety regulations, risk assessments, and occupational health programs aimed at mitigating risks, promoting ergonomic practices, and safeguarding worker well-being.

Climate change represents a contemporary environmental challenge with far-reaching implications for human health. Rising temperatures, extreme weather events, altered precipitation patterns, and shifts in infectious disease dynamics pose complex challenges to public health infrastructure and resilience. Heat-related illnesses, vector-borne diseases, food insecurity, and displacement exacerbate vulnerabilities, underscoring the need for adaptive strategies, sustainable development practices, and global cooperation to mitigate climate-related health risks.

In conclusion, environmental factors exert profound influences on human health, necessitating integrated approaches that address air and water quality, occupational safety, and climate resilience. By prioritizing environmental stewardship, adopting evidence-based policies, and fostering multidisciplinary collaborations, stakeholders can mitigate environmental health risks, promote sustainable development, and safeguard population health for current and future generations.

CHAPTER THREE

Early detection and screening

IMPORTANCE

The importance of early detection in the context of cancer cannot be overstated, serving as a fundamental pillar in the continuum of cancer care and management. Timely detection significantly enhances treatment options, prognosis, and overall survival rates for individuals affected by various forms of cancer. Several key aspects underscore the criticality of early detection:

1. Improved Treatment Outcomes: Detecting cancer in its early stages often allows for less invasive treatment options such as surgery or localized therapies. This

can reduce the need for extensive procedures or aggressive treatments that may be required if the cancer progresses undetected to advanced stages. For example, early-stage breast cancer detected through mammography may only require surgery and possibly radiation therapy, leading to higher cure rates and lower morbidity compared to advanced-stage cancers that may necessitate chemotherapy or more extensive surgeries.

2. Enhanced Survival Rates: Statistics consistently show that cancers detected early are associated with higher survival rates. For many types of cancer, the prognosis improves significantly when the disease is diagnosed and treated before it spreads to other parts of the body. This underscores the critical window of opportunity that early detection provides, where interventions can be more effective in halting or eradicating the disease.

3. Reduced Treatment Costs: Early detection not only improves health outcomes but also contributes to cost savings within healthcare systems. By identifying cancers at an earlier stage, healthcare providers can employ less costly treatment modalities and avoid the substantial financial burden associated with advanced cancer care, including prolonged hospitalizations, intensive therapies, and supportive care needs.

4. Quality of Life: Early detection can preserve quality of life by minimizing the physical, emotional, and social impact of cancer and its treatment. Early-stage cancers often entail less aggressive treatments with fewer side effects, allowing individuals to maintain their daily routines and activities more effectively than those undergoing treatments for advanced-stage disease.

5. Empowerment through Knowledge:

Screening programs and early detection initiatives empower individuals to take proactive steps in managing their health. By knowing their cancer risk and undergoing recommended screenings, individuals can make informed decisions about lifestyle modifications, screening intervals, and preventive measures that may further reduce their cancer risk.

In conclusion, early detection of cancer remains a cornerstone of effective cancer control strategies worldwide. It not only enhances treatment options and survival rates but also reduces healthcare costs and improves the overall quality of life for individuals and their families. Emphasizing the importance of early detection through education, screening programs, and healthcare policy initiatives is essential to further reducing the global burden of cancer.

Common screening tests

Common screening tests for cancer are vital tools in the early detection and prevention of various types of malignancies. These tests are designed to identify abnormalities or precancerous conditions before symptoms develop, allowing for timely intervention and improved treatment outcomes. Here are further details on some of the most widely used screening tests:

1. **Mammography:**

   - Purpose: Mammograms use low-dose X-rays to create detailed images of the breast tissue. They are primarily used for breast cancer screening.

   - Recommendations: For women at average risk, regular mammograms are recommended starting at age 40. Frequency may vary based on individual risk factors, with guidelines suggesting screening every

1-2 years.

- Benefits: Mammography can detect breast cancer early when it is most treatable, often before physical symptoms are noticeable. This allows for less invasive treatment options and higher survival rates.

2. **Pap Smear (Pap Test):**

- Purpose: Pap smears involve collecting cells from the cervix to detect precancerous changes or cervical cancer.

- Recommendations: Typically, screening begins at age 21 and continues at regular intervals (every 3 years for women aged 21-29, every 5 years with HPV testing for women aged 30-65) depending on previous results and risk factors.

- Benefits: Pap smears have been instrumental in reducing cervical cancer incidence and mortality by identifying abnormal cells early, enabling timely treatment and intervention.

3. **Colonoscopy:**

- Purpose: Colonoscopies allow for the direct visualization of the colon and rectum to detect colorectal cancer and precancerous polyps.

- Recommendations: Screening usually starts at age 50 for average-risk individuals, with follow-up screenings every 10 years if no abnormalities are found. Screening intervals may be more frequent for those with a family history of colorectal cancer or other risk factors.

- Benefits: Early detection through colonoscopy can lead to the removal of precancerous polyps before they become cancerous, thereby reducing colorectal cancer incidence and mortality.

4. **Prostate-Specific Antigen (PSA) Test:**

   - Purpose: The PSA test measures levels of a protein produced by the prostate gland. Elevated PSA levels may indicate prostate cancer or other prostate conditions.

   - Recommendations: Guidelines vary, but generally recommend discussing the benefits and risks of PSA screening with healthcare providers, especially for men aged 50 and older or those at higher risk.

   - Benefits: PSA testing can aid in the early detection of prostate cancer, allowing for prompt diagnosis and treatment decisions that may improve outcomes.

5. **Skin Examinations:**

   - Purpose: Regular skin examinations by healthcare providers or self-examinations help detect skin cancers such as melanoma and basal cell carcinoma.

- Recommendations: Individuals are encouraged to perform monthly self-examinations of their skin and seek professional evaluation for any suspicious moles or lesions.

- Benefits: Early detection of skin cancer allows for simpler and less invasive treatment options, often resulting in better outcomes and survival rates.

These screening tests are essential components of comprehensive cancer prevention and control strategies. They empower individuals and healthcare providers to detect cancer at its earliest stages when treatment is most effective, ultimately reducing cancer-related morbidity and mortality. Regular adherence to recommended screening guidelines tailored to individual risk profiles remains critical in maximizing the benefits of these tests.

GUIDELINES FOR SCREENING

Guidelines for cancer screening are pivotal for tailoring interventions to individual risk profiles, ensuring they are both effective and appropriate. These guidelines meticulously consider age and specific risk factors to optimize the timing and frequency of screenings. Here's a comprehensive exploration focusing on age and risk-based guidelines for various types of cancer:

Breast Cancer Screening:

- Age Guidelines: Mammography screening typically begins at age 40 for women at average risk, continuing annually or biennially thereafter. Variations may occur based on individual risk profiles.

- Risk Guidelines: Women with a strong family history of breast cancer or genetic mutations (e.g., BRCA1/BRCA2) should start screening earlier and consider supplementary MRI screenings alongside mammography.

Cervical Cancer Screening:

- Age Guidelines: Pap smears generally commence at age 21 and continue at intervals determined by previous results and HPV co-testing.

- Risk Guidelines: Women with abnormal Pap smear results, a history of cervical intraepithelial neoplasia (CIN) treatment, or HPV infection may require more frequent screenings.

Colorectal Cancer Screening:

- Age Guidelines: Screening starts at age 50 for average-risk individuals, often with colonoscopy every 10 years. Other options include stool-based tests and sigmoidoscopy.

- Risk Guidelines: Those with a family history of colorectal cancer or polyps, inflammatory bowel disease (IBD), or genetic syndromes (e.g., Lynch syndrome) may need earlier or more frequent screenings.

Prostate Cancer Screening:

- Age Guidelines: PSA testing for prostate cancer is typically based on shared decision-making, generally starting around age 50 for average-risk men.

- Risk Guidelines: African American men and those with a family history of prostate cancer may consider starting discussions earlier, around age 45.

Lung Cancer Screening:

- Age Guidelines: Low-dose CT scans are recommended for adults aged 50-80 with a significant smoking history who currently smoke or quit within the past 15 years.

- Risk Guidelines: Individuals with occupational exposure to carcinogens or a personal history of lung cancer may benefit from earlier or more frequent screenings.

Skin Cancer Screening:

- Age Guidelines: Regular skin examinations are beneficial for individuals of all ages, especially those with a history of significant sun exposure or a family history of melanoma.

- Risk Guidelines: People with numerous moles, atypical moles, or a personal history of skin cancer should undergo more frequent skin checks and self-examinations.

General Considerations:

- Shared Decision-Making: Discussions between individuals and healthcare providers are essential for balancing potential benefits and harms, particularly for prostate and lung cancer screenings.

- Individualized Approach: Screening guidelines evolve based on emerging evidence and personalized risk assessments, highlighting the role of healthcare providers in tailoring plans to each patient's unique circumstances.

Adhering to these age and risk-based screening guidelines empowers individuals to take proactive steps in managing their health, facilitating early detection and timely intervention to improve treatment outcomes and overall health outcomes.

CHAPTER FOUR

Immunization Against Cancer

Role of vaccines in preventing cancer

In contemporary oncology, the role of vaccines stands pivotal in the prevention of cancer, notably exemplified through vaccines targeting Human Papillomavirus (HPV) and Hepatitis B virus. These vaccinations serve as profound advancements in medical science, showcasing their capability to mitigate the incidence of virally-induced cancers.

In the realm of cancer prevention, vaccines targeting Human Papillomavirus (HPV) and Hepatitis B virus play indispensable roles, offering profound contributions to public health strategies worldwide.

HPV vaccines are particularly notable for

their ability to prevent infections by high-risk HPV types known to cause a spectrum of cancers, including cervical, anal, vulvar, vaginal, penile, and oropharyngeal cancers. By targeting these viral strains early in life, before individuals become sexually active, HPV vaccines effectively reduce the likelihood of HPV-related malignancies. The success of these vaccines lies not only in their ability to prevent initial infections but also in their potential to decrease the prevalence of HPV within populations over time, thereby indirectly reducing the incidence of associated cancers.

Similarly, Hepatitis B vaccines have demonstrated significant impact in preventing liver cancer, which is often linked to chronic Hepatitis B virus infection. By immunizing individuals against Hepatitis B early in infancy or during adolescence, these vaccines substantially decrease the risk of developing chronic Hepatitis B infection and subsequently lower the long-term risk of liver cancer. This preventive approach underscores the critical role of vaccination in interrupting the chain of events leading to cancer development.

Moreover, beyond individual benefits, widespread vaccination against HPV and Hepatitis B contributes to broader public health goals by reducing the overall burden of these cancers. By preventing infections that can lead to cancerous transformations, these vaccines not only protect vaccinated individuals but also contribute to herd immunity, indirectly shielding unvaccinated individuals from potential exposure to these viruses.

In essence, the role of HPV and Hepatitis B vaccines in cancer prevention extends beyond individual protection to encompass community-wide health benefits. Their integration into national immunization programs represents a pivotal stride in reducing the global burden of cancer, emphasizing the critical intersection of vaccination and oncological prevention strategies.

Cancer vaccines, particularly those targeting viruses like HPV and Hepatitis B, offer significant benefits in the realm of disease prevention, but they also present several notable limitations.

Benefits of cancer vaccines

1. Preventive Efficacy: Cancer vaccines, such as those against HPV and Hepatitis B, have demonstrated high efficacy in preventing infections that are strongly linked to cancer development. For instance, HPV vaccines have been shown to be highly effective in preventing cervical cancer and other HPV-related cancers by targeting the viral strains responsible for these malignancies.

2. Population-wide Impact: By reducing the prevalence of viral infections known to cause cancer, vaccines contribute to a decrease in the overall incidence of associated malignancies within populations. This population-wide impact is particularly significant in public health efforts to control and reduce the burden of certain types of cancer.

3. Long-term Protection: Vaccination against HPV and Hepatitis B provides long-term protection against viral infections that can lead to cancer, offering individuals immunity early in life and potentially throughout their lifetime. This long-term protection is crucial in preventing chronic infections that may progress to cancer over time.

4. Herd Immunity: High vaccination coverage can lead to herd immunity, where the overall transmission of the virus is reduced in the population. This indirectly

protects individuals who are not vaccinated or who may not develop strong immune responses to vaccination, thus further lowering the risk of cancer transmission.

5. Cost-effectiveness: Despite initial costs associated with vaccine development and distribution, cancer vaccines are generally considered cost-effective over the long term. They reduce the economic burden of treating cancers that could have been prevented through vaccination, including costs related to healthcare, lost productivity, and quality of life.

Limitations of cancer vaccines

1. Incomplete Coverage: Cancer vaccines may not provide protection against all strains of a virus or all types of cancers associated with that virus. For example, current HPV vaccines primarily target the most common high-risk HPV types, but

there are other less common types that can also cause cancer.

2. Vaccine Hesitancy: Public acceptance and uptake of cancer vaccines can be influenced by various factors, including misinformation, concerns about safety, and cultural or religious beliefs. Vaccine hesitancy can limit the effectiveness of vaccination programs in achieving high coverage rates needed for herd immunity.

3. Viral Strain Variability: Viruses like HPV can exhibit genetic variability, leading to different strains with varying degrees of oncogenic potential. Vaccine efficacy may be affected if new viral strains emerge that are not covered by existing vaccines.

4. Logistical Challenges: Distribution and administration of vaccines, especially in resource-limited settings or regions with weak healthcare infrastructure, pose logistical challenges. Maintaining the cold chain for vaccine storage and ensuring

access to remote or underserved populations can be barriers to achieving high vaccination coverage.

5. Complexity of Cancer Biology: Cancer development involves complex interactions between genetic, environmental, and immune factors. Vaccines targeting viral infections associated with cancer address only one aspect of cancer prevention and may not be effective against cancers with non-viral origins or those influenced by multiple risk factors.

In conclusion, while cancer vaccines offer substantial benefits in preventing virus-associated cancers and reducing disease burden, addressing their limitations requires ongoing research, education, and healthcare infrastructure development to optimize their effectiveness and accessibility globally.

CHAPTER FIVE

Diet and Nutrition

In this chapter, we explore the profound influence of dietary choices on the incidence of cancer. We delve into the specific ways in which various diets can either mitigate or exacerbate cancer risk. Furthermore, we examine the role of key nutrients and foods renowned for their potential anti-cancer properties, such as antioxidants and dietary fiber. Additionally, comprehensive dietary guidelines tailored specifically for the prevention of cancer are meticulously analyzed and discussed, offering invaluable insights into optimizing nutritional strategies for health promotion and disease prevention.

IMPACT OF DIET ON CANCER RISK

The impact of diet on cancer risk is a multifaceted subject of profound scientific interest and public health importance. Extensive research has consistently demonstrated that dietary habits play a pivotal role in influencing the likelihood of developing various types of cancer.

Certain dietary patterns, such as diets high in processed meats, sugary beverages, and refined carbohydrates, have been linked to an increased risk of cancers including colorectal, breast, and prostate cancers. Conversely, diets rich in fruits, vegetables, whole grains, and lean proteins have been associated with a lower incidence of cancer.

Several mechanisms underline the relationship between diet and cancer risk. For instance, high consumption of red and processed meats is thought to contribute to cancer risk through mechanisms involving heterocyclic amines, polycyclic aromatic hydrocarbons, and N-nitroso compounds formed during cooking and processing. On the other hand, diets rich in fruits and vegetables provide essential vitamins, minerals, and phytochemicals with antioxidant and anti-inflammatory properties, which help protect cells from damage that can lead to cancer.

Moreover, dietary factors influence obesity, insulin resistance, and chronic inflammation, all of which are known contributors to cancer development. Maintaining a healthy weight through balanced nutrition and regular physical activity is therefore crucial in reducing cancer risk.

In summary, the impact of diet on cancer risk underscores the importance of adopting a balanced and nutrient-rich diet as a fundamental strategy in cancer prevention. Understanding these relationships empowers individuals and healthcare providers alike to make informed dietary choices that promote long-term health and well-being.

ANTI-CANCER FOODS AND NUTRIENTS

Anti-cancer foods and nutrients, such as antioxidants and dietary fiber, are pivotal in the realm of cancer prevention and overall health maintenance. Antioxidants, including vitamins C and E, beta-carotene, and selenium, play a crucial role in neutralizing free radicals—unstable molecules that can damage cells and potentially lead to cancerous changes. These compounds are abundantly found in various fruits (e.g., berries, citrus fruits), vegetables (e.g., spinach, kale), nuts, seeds, and whole grains. By scavenging free radicals, antioxidants help protect cellular DNA and prevent mutations that could initiate cancer development.

Dietary fiber, another cornerstone of anti-cancer nutrition, encompasses both soluble and insoluble forms found in foods like whole grains, legumes, fruits, and vegetables. Soluble fiber, such as that found in oats and apples, helps regulate blood sugar levels and cholesterol, thereby reducing the risk of obesity and associated cancers. Insoluble fiber, prevalent in wheat bran and vegetables, aids in maintaining bowel regularity and preventing colorectal cancer by speeding up the elimination of carcinogens and promoting a healthy gut microbiome.

Moreover, the synergistic effects of antioxidants and fiber contribute to overall health benefits beyond cancer prevention. For instance, a diet rich in these nutrients supports cardiovascular health, enhances immune function, and promotes optimal digestion—all crucial components of a holistic approach to well-being.

Incorporating a diverse array of anti-cancer foods into daily meals not only ensures a broad spectrum of protective nutrients but also cultivates sustainable dietary habits that promote long-term health. By emphasizing whole, minimally processed foods and adopting a balanced diet, individuals can harness the potential of antioxidants and fiber to mitigate cancer risk and enhance overall quality of life.

DIETARY GUIDELINES FOR CANCER PREVENTION

Dietary guidelines aimed at cancer prevention are grounded in evidence-based recommendations that emphasize the importance of a balanced and varied diet. These guidelines serve as a proactive approach to reducing cancer risk through nutritional strategies:

1. Emphasize Plant-Based Foods: Base your diet on a variety of fruits, vegetables, whole grains, legumes, and nuts. These foods are rich in vitamins, minerals, antioxidants, and dietary fiber, which collectively support immune function and protect against cellular damage that can lead to cancer.

2. Limit Red and Processed Meats: Minimize consumption of red meats (e.g., beef, pork, lamb) and processed meats (e.g., bacon, sausage, deli meats), which have been linked to an increased risk of colorectal and other cancers. When consuming meat, opt for lean cuts and smaller portions.

3. Choose Healthy Fats: Replace saturated and trans fats with healthier fats found in olive oil, avocados, nuts, and seeds. These fats support heart health and provide essential nutrients without contributing to cancer risk.

4. Reduce Sugar and Refined Carbohydrates: Limit foods and beverages high in added sugars and refined carbohydrates, as they can contribute to obesity and inflammation, both of which are linked to an increased risk of cancer.

5. Moderate Alcohol Consumption: If you drink alcohol, do so in moderation. Alcohol consumption has been associated with an increased risk of several cancers, including breast, liver, and colorectal cancers. The recommended limit is up to one drink per day for women and up to two drinks per day for men.

6. Be Mindful of Portions and Overall Caloric Intake: Maintain a healthy weight through balanced portion sizes and regular physical activity. Excess body weight, especially abdominal fat, is a risk factor for multiple types of cancer.

7. Stay Hydrated: Drink plenty of water throughout the day. Water supports overall

health and helps maintain proper bodily functions, including digestion and elimination of toxins.

8. Limit Sodium and Processed Foods: Reduce intake of foods high in salt and processed foods, which may contribute to an increased risk of stomach cancer and other health issues.

9. Follow Food Safety Practices: Handle, cook, and store foods properly to prevent foodborne illnesses, which can weaken the immune system and potentially increase cancer risk.

10. Maintain a Healthy Lifestyle: In addition to diet, incorporate regular physical activity and avoid tobacco in any form to further reduce cancer risk.

By adhering to these dietary guidelines and adopting a lifestyle that prioritizes health-promoting behaviors, individuals can significantly enhance their resilience against cancer and improve overall well-being.

CHAPTER SIX

Physical Activity and Cancer Prevention

In this chapter, the profound impact of exercise on mitigating cancer risk is explored. The discussion begins by outlining the multifaceted benefits associated with regular physical activity, including its role in lowering the likelihood of developing various types of cancer. Furthermore, the chapter delineates the recommended levels of physical activity deemed optimal for reducing cancer incidence, providing a comprehensive framework supported by current research and guidelines.

Moreover, the chapter delves into tailored exercise strategies specifically designed for cancer survivors. These strategies encompass a spectrum of physical activities tailored to the unique needs and conditions of individuals post-treatment. By addressing these strategies, the chapter aims to empower survivors with practical approaches to enhance their overall well-being and quality of life.

Through an in-depth exploration of these themes, this chapter underscores the pivotal role of physical activity not only in cancer prevention but also in fostering resilience and recovery among those affected by cancer.

BENEFITS OF EXERCISE IN REDUCING CANCER RISK

Regular physical activity confers a multitude of benefits that significantly contribute to reducing the risk of cancer. Firstly, engaging in exercise helps to maintain a healthy body weight, thereby lowering the likelihood of obesity, a known risk factor for various cancers such as breast, colon, and endometrial cancers. Furthermore, physical activity plays a crucial role in modulating hormone levels, such as reducing estrogen and insulin, which are linked to the development and progression of certain cancers.

Moreover, exercise enhances immune function and promotes efficient circulation, both of which are critical in suppressing tumor growth and improving overall health resilience against cancerous cells. Additionally, regular physical activity is associated with reducing chronic inflammation in the body, which is a common precursor to many types of cancer.

Beyond these physiological benefits, exercise also contributes to psychological well-being, reducing stress, anxiety, and depression, which are conditions that can indirectly influence cancer risk through their impact on immune function and overall health.

By emphasizing these diverse mechanisms, it becomes evident that integrating regular physical activity into daily routines not only promotes physical fitness but also serves as a potent preventive measure against cancer, underscoring its indispensable role in public health strategies aimed at cancer prevention and management.

RECOMMENDED LEVELS OF PHYSICAL ACTIVITY

The recommended suitable exercises for cancer prevention and management vary depending on individual health conditions, fitness levels, and treatment history. Generally, a combination of aerobic, strength training, and flexibility exercises is beneficial:

1. Aerobic Exercise: Activities such as walking, jogging, cycling, swimming, or dancing help improve cardiovascular

fitness, boost immune function, and aid in weight management. Aim for at least 150 minutes of moderate-intensity aerobic exercise per week, or 75 minutes of vigorous-intensity exercise spread throughout the week.

2. Strength Training: This includes exercises using weights, resistance bands, or body weight (e.g., squats, lunges, push-ups). Strength training helps maintain muscle mass, bone density, and overall strength, which is crucial during and after cancer treatment.

3. Flexibility and Stretching: Incorporate exercises that improve flexibility and range of motion, such as yoga or Pilates. These activities can help reduce muscle tension, improve posture, and enhance relaxation.

4. Balance Exercises: Especially important for older adults or those at risk of falls due to treatment side effects or aging. Balance exercises can include standing on one foot,

heel-to-toe walking, or Tai Chi.

5. Mind-Body Exercises: Practices like yoga, Tai Chi, or meditation can help reduce stress, improve mood, and enhance overall well-being. These exercises also promote relaxation and mindfulness, which can be beneficial during cancer treatment and recovery.

It's crucial to consult with healthcare providers or qualified exercise professionals before starting any new exercise regimen, especially for individuals undergoing cancer treatment or recovery. They can provide personalized recommendations based on individual needs and health status to ensure safe and effective exercise participation.

Exercise Strategies for Cancer Survivors

1. **Types of Exercise:**

   - Aerobic Exercise: Engage in activities like

walking, jogging, cycling, or swimming to improve cardiovascular fitness. Start with low intensity and gradually increase duration and intensity as tolerated.

- Strength Training: Incorporate resistance exercises using body weight, resistance bands, or light weights to build muscle strength. Focus on major muscle groups (legs, arms, back, abdomen) and aim for 2-3 sessions per week.

- Flexibility and Balance: Include stretching exercises to improve flexibility and balance, which can help reduce stiffness and prevent falls. Practices like yoga or tai chi are beneficial for enhancing both flexibility and balance.

2. **Safety Considerations:**

- Consultation with Healthcare Team: Always consult with your oncologist or healthcare provider before starting any exercise program. They can provide personalized recommendations based on your specific cancer type, treatment history, and current health status.

   - Monitor Symptoms: Pay attention to how your body responds to exercise. It's normal to experience fatigue, but severe or unusual symptoms such as pain, dizziness, or shortness of breath should prompt you to stop and consult your healthcare provider.

   - Adaptations for Side Effects: Modify exercises based on any lingering side effects of cancer treatment. For example, if you have lymphedema, avoid heavy lifting or activities that put strain on affected limbs.

3. **Psychosocial Benefits:**

   - Enhanced Mood and Well-being: Regular physical activity can improve mood, reduce anxiety and depression, and enhance overall quality of life. It provides a positive outlet for managing stress associated with cancer survivorship.

- Social Support: Joining exercise classes or groups specifically designed for cancer survivors can provide a supportive environment where you can connect with others who understand your experience.

4. **Integration into Daily Routine:**

- Set Realistic Goals: Establish achievable exercise goals that fit into your daily routine. This could be as simple as taking short walks during breaks or engaging in gentle stretching before bedtime.

- Gradual Progression: Start with shorter durations and lower intensities, then gradually increase both as your fitness improves and you feel comfortable.

5. **Long-Term Benefits:**

- Reduced Risk of Recurrence: Some studies suggest that regular physical activity may reduce the risk of cancer recurrence and improve survival rates for certain cancer types. However, more research is needed in this area.

- Overall Health Improvement: Exercise promotes cardiovascular health, maintains muscle mass and bone density, and can help manage weight, all of which contribute to overall health and well-being.

6. **Incorporating Mindfulness and Relaxation Techniques:**

- Breathing Exercises: Practice deep breathing exercises or mindfulness techniques before, during, or after exercise to promote relaxation and reduce stress.

- Mind-Body Practices: Incorporate mind-body practices such as meditation, guided imagery, or progressive muscle relaxation to complement your physical activity routine.

7. **Long-Term Maintenance:**

- Lifestyle Integration: Aim to integrate physical activity as a lifelong habit. Find activities you enjoy and can sustain over time, adjusting as needed to accommodate changes in your health or energy levels.

- Regular Monitoring: Continue to monitor your physical activity levels and adjust your routine as necessary to maintain fitness and address any new health considerations that may arise.

By tailoring exercise strategies to individual needs and capabilities, cancer survivors can benefit greatly from physical activity in enhancing their physical, emotional, and social well-being during and after cancer treatment. Always prioritize safety and consult healthcare professionals for guidance throughout your exercise journey.

CHAPTER SEVEN

Smoking Cessation

Link between Smoking and Cancer

Smoking is intricately linked to various types of cancer, including lung, throat, mouth, and esophageal cancers. The harmful chemicals in tobacco smoke damage DNA and lead to mutations that can result in cancerous growths. Understanding this link is crucial for motivating individuals to quit smoking and for policymakers to implement effective public health measures.

This is well-established and deeply concerning due to the multitude of harmful chemicals present in tobacco smoke. Here are further details on this critical connection:

1. Carcinogens in Tobacco Smoke:

- Tobacco smoke contains over 7,000 chemicals, including at least 70 known carcinogens (substances capable of causing cancer).

- Carcinogens like benzene, formaldehyde, and polycyclic aromatic hydrocarbons (PAHs) are formed during the combustion of tobacco and are directly responsible for damaging DNA.

2. Impact on Cellular Level:

- The chemicals in tobacco smoke enter the bloodstream and reach nearly every organ in the body.

- When these chemicals interact with DNA in cells, they cause mutations that disrupt normal cell growth and division processes.

- Over time, accumulated genetic mutations can lead to the uncontrolled growth of cancerous cells.

3. Secondhand Smoke and Cancer Risk:

- Secondhand smoke, which is the combination of smoke from the burning end of a cigarette and smoke exhaled by the smoker, also contains carcinogens.

- Non-smokers exposed to secondhand smoke have an increased risk of developing lung cancer and other respiratory conditions.

4. Global Health Impact:

- Smoking-related cancers are a significant public health concern globally, contributing to millions of deaths annually.

- Efforts to reduce smoking prevalence

through tobacco control policies, public health campaigns, and smoking cessation programs are crucial to mitigating the burden of cancer and other smoking-related diseases.

Types of Cancer Linked to Smoking

1.   - Lung Cancer: Smoking is the primary cause of lung cancer, accounting for approximately 85% of cases in the United States. The risk of lung cancer increases with the duration and intensity of smoking.

2.   - Other Respiratory Cancers: Smoking is also linked to cancers of the throat, mouth, nasal cavity, sinuses, larynx (voice box), and trachea (windpipe).

3.   - Gastrointestinal Cancers: Smoking increases the risk of cancers of the esophagus, stomach, pancreas, and colon.

=>   - Other Types: Tobacco use is

associated with an increased risk of cancers in organs not directly exposed to tobacco smoke, such as the bladder and cervix, due to systemic effects and carcinogen exposure.

Understanding the detailed mechanisms by which smoking contributes to cancer underscores the urgency of promoting smoking cessation and implementing effective tobacco control measures. Efforts to reduce smoking rates can significantly reduce the incidence of smoking-related cancers and improve public health outcomes worldwide.

methods and resources for quitting smoking:

1. Behavioral Support and Counseling:

- Individual Counseling: One-on-one sessions with trained counselors or therapists can help smokers identify triggers, develop coping strategies, and set realistic goals for quitting.

- Group Counseling: Support groups provide a sense of community and shared experience, offering encouragement, motivation, and accountability.

- Telephone Quitlines: Many countries operate quitlines staffed by counselors who provide personalized advice, support, and information about cessation resources.

2. Medications for Smoking Cessation:

- Nicotine Replacement Therapy (NRT): Available in various forms such as patches, gums, lozenges, inhalers, and nasal sprays. NRT helps reduce withdrawal symptoms by providing controlled doses of nicotine without the harmful chemicals found in tobacco smoke.

- Prescription Medications: Drugs like

bupropion (Zyban) and varenicline (Chantix/Champix) can reduce cravings and withdrawal symptoms by altering brain chemistry. These medications are available by prescription and are typically used under medical supervision.

3. Digital and Mobile Resources:

- Mobile Apps: There are numerous smartphone apps designed to assist smokers in quitting. These apps often include features such as tracking progress, setting goals, providing motivational messages, and offering tips to manage cravings and stress.

- Online Programs: Web-based cessation programs offer interactive tools, educational resources, and forums for peer support. They may also provide personalized quitting plans based on individual smoking habits and preferences.

4. Alternative Therapies and Techniques:

- Mindfulness and Meditation: Practices like mindfulness-based stress reduction (MBSR) or meditation can help smokers manage stress and cravings more effectively.

- Acupuncture: Some people find acupuncture sessions helpful in reducing nicotine cravings and withdrawal symptoms.

- Hypnosis: Hypnotherapy may assist individuals in changing their behavior and attitudes towards smoking cessation.

5. Community Support and Resources:

- Support Groups: Beyond counseling, support groups (both in-person and online) provide a sense of community, shared experience, and encouragement during the quitting process.

- Community Programs: Local health departments, non-profit organizations, and community centers often offer smoking cessation programs, workshops, and events.

6. Healthcare Provider Support:

- Primary Care Providers: Doctors, nurse practitioners, and other healthcare professionals can provide guidance, prescribe medications, and monitor progress during cessation attempts.

- Specialist Clinics: Some hospitals and clinics specialize in smoking cessation and offer comprehensive services, including medical evaluations, counseling, and access to medications.

Effective smoking cessation often involves a combination of these resources tailored to individual needs and preferences. The availability and utilization of these methods can significantly improve the chances of successfully quitting smoking and maintaining long-term abstinence.

PUBLIC HEALTH STRATEGIES TO REDUCE SMOKING-RELATED CANCERS

These are multifaceted and involve coordinated efforts at various levels of society. These strategies aim to decrease tobacco use prevalence, minimize exposure to secondhand smoke, and promote healthier lifestyles. Here's a detailed exploration of these strategies:

1. Tobacco Control Policies:

 - Tobacco Taxes and Price Increases: Higher taxes on tobacco products make smoking more expensive, reducing affordability and discouraging initiation and continuation of smoking.

- Smoke-Free Laws: Comprehensive smoke-free policies in public places, workplaces, and hospitality venues protect non-smokers from secondhand smoke exposure and encourage smokers to quit.

- Advertising Bans and Restrictions: Prohibiting tobacco advertising, promotion, and sponsorship reduces the visibility and appeal of tobacco products, particularly to youth.

- Packaging and Labeling Regulations: Implementing plain packaging and graphic health warnings on tobacco products effectively communicates the risks of smoking and discourages consumption.

2. Education and Awareness Campaigns:

- Media Campaigns: Public education initiatives using mass media (television, radio, internet, etc.) raise awareness about the health risks of smoking, secondhand smoke exposure, and the benefits of quitting.

- School-Based Programs: Integrating tobacco education into school curricula helps prevent youth initiation by promoting knowledge about the dangers of smoking and enhancing critical thinking skills.

- Community Outreach: Engaging communities through events, workshops, and partnerships with local organizations reinforces messaging and supports smoking cessation efforts.

3. Access to Cessation Services:

- Quitlines: Telephone quitlines provide free counseling, support, and information about quitting smoking. They often connect smokers with resources such as NRT and cessation clinics.

-    Healthcare Provider Support: Encouraging healthcare professionals to routinely screen for tobacco use, offer brief cessation advice, and provide medications or referrals to specialized cessation services.

- Pharmacotherapy Coverage: Ensuring affordable access to medications (e.g., NRT, bupropion, varenicline) through healthcare coverage and subsidies increases utilization and effectiveness of cessation treatments.

4. Support for Smoke-Free Environments:

- Workplace Initiatives: Promoting smoke-free workplaces through policies, employee cessation programs, and cessation support resources improves employee health and productivity.

- Public Spaces and Housing: Advocating for and implementing smoke-free policies in public parks, beaches, multi-unit housing, and vehicles reduces exposure to secondhand smoke and supports smoke-free norms.

5. Research and Surveillance:

- Surveillance Systems: Monitoring tobacco use prevalence, smoking behaviors, and trends in tobacco-related diseases provides data for evaluating interventions and guiding policy decisions.

- Research Funding: Investing in research on smoking cessation strategies, tobacco control policies, and the health impacts of smoking facilitates evidence-based policymaking and program development.

6. Global Collaboration and Advocacy:

- International Treaties and Agreements: Supporting and implementing provisions of the WHO Framework Convention on Tobacco Control (FCTC) strengthens global efforts to reduce tobacco use and its health consequences.

- Advocacy and Coalition Building: Collaborating with international, national, and local stakeholders, including governments, non-governmental organizations (NGOs), and advocacy groups, amplifies efforts to enact and enforce effective tobacco control measures.

These public health strategies work synergistically to create environments that support tobacco-free living, reduce smoking-related cancers, and improve overall public health. Effective implementation requires sustained commitment, resources, and collaboration across sectors to achieve lasting reductions

in tobacco use and its associated health
burdens.

CHAPTER EIGHT

Environmental and occupational exposures

Carcinogens in the environment and workplace

- Chemicals: This includes substances like asbestos, benzene, formaldehyde, and various industrial solvents which have been conclusively linked to cancer through epidemiological studies and toxicological research.

- Radiation: Sources such as ionizing radiation (e.g., from X-rays, radioactive isotopes) and ultraviolet (UV) radiation (from sunlight and artificial sources) are known to increase cancer risk.

- Biological Agents: Certain viruses (e.g., hepatitis B and C viruses, human papillomavirus) and bacteria (e.g., Helicobacter pylori) are recognized carcinogens.

- Other Hazards: Environmental factors like air pollution (e.g., particulate matter, polycyclic aromatic hydrocarbons) and dietary factors (e.g., aflatoxins in moldy foods) can also contribute to cancer risk.

Regulations and Safety Measures to reduce exposure

- Government Regulations: National and international agencies (e.g., OSHA in the United States, EU directives) set permissible exposure limits (PELs) and guidelines for handling carcinogens in workplaces.

- Workplace Safety Protocols: Employers are required to implement engineering controls (ventilation systems, enclosure of hazardous processes), administrative controls (workplace policies, training programs), and personal protective equipment (respirators, gloves) to minimize exposure.

- International Standards: Organizations like the International Agency for Research on Cancer (IARC) classify carcinogens and provide scientific evidence to inform regulatory decisions worldwide.

Case Studies of occupational cancer risk

- Occupational Cancer Risks: Examples may include studies on lung cancer among asbestos miners, mesothelioma in construction workers exposed to asbestos, and leukemia among workers exposed to benzene in the petrochemical industry.

- Epidemiological Evidence: These studies typically involve long-term monitoring of exposed populations to assess cancer incidence rates compared to unexposed or minimally exposed groups.

- Legal and Regulatory Responses: High-profile cases, such as litigation against companies for failing to protect workers from carcinogenic exposures, highlight the need for stringent regulations and accountability.

Preventive Strategies

1. Engineering Controls: Designing and implementing processes and technologies to eliminate or reduce exposure to carcinogens at the source (e.g., substitution of hazardous chemicals with safer alternatives).

2. Personal Protective Equipment (PPE): Ensuring workers have access to and properly use PPE such as respirators, gloves, and protective clothing.

3. Training and Education: Providing comprehensive training on the risks associated with carcinogens, safe handling

procedures, and the importance of hygiene practices (e.g., washing hands after handling hazardous materials).

Public Health Implications

(a).   Health   Surveillance: Monitoring exposed populations for early detection of cancer and other health effects, allowing for timely intervention and treatment.

(b). Policy Advocacy: Supporting policies that strengthen regulatory frameworks, increase funding for research on occupational cancer, and improve access to healthcare for affected workers.

 (c). Community Awareness: Educating communities living near industrial sites about potential environmental exposures and advocating for measures to reduce pollution and protect public health.

In summary, Chapter 8 provides a detailed exploration of the multifaceted issues surrounding environmental and occupational exposures to carcinogens, emphasizing both the scientific evidence of risks and the practical strategies to mitigate these risks and safeguard human health.

CHAPTER NINE

Psychological and Social Aspects of Cancer

IMPACT OF STRESS AND MENTAL HEALTH ON CANCER PREVENTION

The impact of stress and mental health on cancer prevention is a multifaceted topic that involves understanding how psychological factors can influence biological processes and behaviors that contribute to cancer risk. Here's a more detailed exploration:

1. Psychosocial Factors and Cancer Risk:

   - Immune Function: Chronic stress has been linked to dysregulation of the immune system. Stress hormones like cortisol can suppress immune responses, potentially compromising the body's ability to recognize and destroy cancerous cells.

- Inflammation: Stress can promote chronic inflammation, which is associated with the development and progression of many types of cancer. Inflammatory cytokines and other immune molecules produced during stress may create a microenvironment that supports tumor growth.

- Hormonal Imbalance: Stress hormones such as cortisol and adrenaline can disrupt hormonal balance in the body. For instance, elevated levels of cortisol over time may alter the metabolism of sex hormones (e.g., estrogen, testosterone), which are implicated in certain cancers like breast and prostate cancer.

2. Behavioral Factors Influenced by Mental Health:

- Smoking and Alcohol Use: Individuals

experiencing chronic stress or mental health disorders may be more likely to engage in behaviors like smoking tobacco and consuming alcohol excessively. These behaviors are major risk factors for various cancers, including lung, liver, and oral cancers.

- Diet and Physical Activity: Stress can affect dietary choices, leading to preferences for high-fat or sugary foods that are associated with increased cancer risk. Additionally, stress may contribute to sedentary behaviors and reduced physical activity, which are linked to obesity and higher cancer risk.

3. Psychological Interventions for Cancer Prevention:

- Stress Management Techniques: Techniques such as relaxation exercises, mindfulness meditation, and biofeedback can help individuals reduce stress levels and mitigate its potential impact on cancer risk.

- Cognitive-Behavioral Therapy (CBT): CBT focuses on identifying and changing maladaptive thought patterns and behaviors. It can help individuals develop coping strategies, improve problem-solving skills, and enhance resilience in the face of stressors that may contribute to cancer risk behaviors.

- Promotion of Healthy Lifestyle Choices: Psychological interventions can also promote adherence to healthy lifestyle behaviors such as maintaining a balanced diet, engaging in regular physical activity, and avoiding tobacco and excessive alcohol consumption.

4. Research and Evidence:

- Epidemiological Studies: Longitudinal studies have provided evidence linking chronic stress, psychological distress, and mental health disorders with increased cancer incidence and mortality rates.

- Biological Mechanisms: Advances in understanding the biological pathways through which stress affects cancer risk, including hormonal, immune, and inflammatory processes, are contributing to a deeper understanding of the relationship between mental health and cancer.

5. Public Health Implications:

- Integrated Care Approaches: Recognizing the interplay between mental health and cancer risk underscores the importance of integrated care approaches that address both physical and psychological aspects of health.

- Preventive Strategies: Implementing

population-level strategies to promote mental well-being, reduce chronic stress, and support healthy behaviors can potentially reduce the burden of cancer at a societal level.

In conclusion, addressing the impact of stress and mental health on cancer prevention involves not only understanding the biological mechanisms involved but also implementing effective psychological interventions and promoting healthy behaviors to mitigate cancer risk factors associated with mental distress. This holistic approach is essential for comprehensive cancer prevention and management strategies.

Support networks for cancer patients and survivors

This plays a crucial role in providing

emotional, practical, and informational support throughout the cancer journey. Here's a more detailed exploration of these networks:

1. Family and Social Support:

- Emotional Comfort: Family members, close friends, and caregivers offer emotional support by providing empathy, encouragement, and a sense of reassurance during challenging times. Their presence can help alleviate feelings of isolation and loneliness commonly experienced by cancer patients.

- Practical Assistance: Support networks assist with practical needs such as transportation to medical appointments, help with household chores, and caregiving responsibilities, enabling patients to focus on their treatment and recovery.

- Advocacy and Communication: Family

members and caregivers often serve as advocates for the patient, communicating with healthcare providers, navigating the healthcare system, and ensuring that the patient's preferences and needs are met.

2. Peer Support Groups:

- Shared Experiences: Peer support groups connect individuals who have experienced similar cancer diagnoses, treatments, and challenges. Sharing experiences and stories with others who understand firsthand can provide a profound sense of validation and solidarity.

- Information Sharing: Participants exchange practical advice, insights into treatment options, and coping strategies based on personal experiences, which can supplement information provided by healthcare professionals.

- Emotional Validation: Group members

offer mutual emotional support, empathy, and understanding, creating a safe space for expressing fears, frustrations, and uncertainties without judgment.

3. Professional Support Services:

- Oncology Social Workers: These professionals specialize in providing psychosocial support to cancer patients and their families. They offer counseling, assistance with navigating financial and insurance issues, and access to community resources.

- Psychologists and Counselors: Mental health professionals with expertise in oncology provide individual and group therapy to address emotional distress, anxiety, depression, and adjustment issues related to cancer diagnosis, treatment, and survivorship.

- Supportive Care Programs: Hospitals and

cancer centers often offer structured programs that include educational workshops, wellness activities (e.g., yoga, art therapy), and support groups facilitated by trained professionals to enhance coping skills and promote overall well-being.

4. Online Support Communities:

- Accessibility and Convenience: Virtual support networks, including online forums, social media groups, and telehealth platforms, provide accessible support to individuals who may not have local support group options or who prefer connecting remotely.

- Anonymity and Privacy: Online communities allow individuals to discuss sensitive topics anonymously, facilitating open and honest communication about their experiences, concerns, and emotions related to cancer.

5. Long-Term Support and Survivorship:

- Continued Support Needs: Support networks remain valuable during the transition from active treatment to survivorship, helping individuals navigate ongoing physical, emotional, and social challenges.

- Celebrating Milestones: Peer support groups and social networks celebrate milestones such as treatment milestones, remission, and survivorship anniversaries, reinforcing a sense of hope, resilience, and community among survivors.

Overall, support networks for cancer patients and survivors encompass a wide range of interpersonal connections, professional services, and community resources that collectively contribute to improved quality of life, emotional well-being, and resilience throughout the cancer journey and beyond. These networks highlight the importance of holistic care approaches that address not only medical needs but also psychosocial aspects of cancer care.

Coping strategies and resilience-building techniques

These are essential for individuals facing the challenges of cancer diagnosis, treatment, and survivorship. These approaches empower patients and survivors to navigate the emotional, physical, and practical aspects of their journey with strength and adaptability. Here's a more detailed exploration:

1. Adaptive Coping Skills:

   - Problem-Solving: Encourages patients to identify specific challenges related to their diagnosis or treatment and develop practical strategies to address them. This approach fosters a sense of control and empowerment over their circumstances.

- Positive Reframing: Involves finding meaning, growth, or opportunities for personal development in the face of adversity. It helps individuals shift their perspective from focusing solely on difficulties to recognizing potential positives and opportunities for learning and resilience.

- Acceptance and Mindfulness: Emphasizes acknowledging and accepting one's thoughts, emotions, and circumstances without judgment. Mindfulness practices, such as meditation and deep breathing exercises, can help reduce stress, enhance emotional regulation, and improve overall well-being.

2. Resilience Factors:

- Optimism and Hope: Maintaining a positive outlook and belief in the possibility of recovery and improvement can enhance resilience. Optimistic individuals tend to perceive setbacks as temporary and manageable, which supports their ability to cope effectively with challenges.

- Social Support Networks: Building and maintaining strong connections with family, friends, and supportive peers provides emotional validation, practical assistance, and a sense of belonging. These relationships serve as a buffer against stress and promote resilience during difficult times.

- Spirituality and Meaning-Making: Drawing on spiritual beliefs, values, or a sense of purpose can provide individuals with inner strength, comfort, and guidance. Engaging in activities that align with personal values and beliefs can contribute to a sense of meaning and resilience.

3. Interventions and Programs:

- Resilience Training Programs: Structured programs offer evidence-based strategies and skills training to enhance resilience. These may include cognitive-behavioral interventions, psychoeducation workshops, and resilience-building exercises tailored to the needs of cancer patients and survivors.

- Psychotherapy and Counseling: Individual or group therapy sessions with psychologists or counselors specializing in oncology provide a safe space to explore and process emotions, develop coping strategies, and strengthen resilience.

- Holistic and Integrative Therapies: Complementary therapies such as art therapy, music therapy, yoga, and acupuncture can complement medical treatment by promoting relaxation, reducing anxiety, and fostering emotional expression and resilience.

4. Personal Growth and Adaptation:

   - Learning and Adapting: Encourages individuals to learn from their experiences, adapt to changing circumstances, and develop new skills or perspectives that contribute to personal growth and resilience.

   - Setting Realistic Goals: Establishing achievable goals, both short-term and long-term, provides a sense of purpose and direction. Celebrating milestones and accomplishments along the way reinforces motivation and resilience.

   - Self-Care Practices: Prioritizing self-care activities, such as adequate rest, nutrition, physical activity, and hobbies that bring joy and relaxation, supports overall well-being and resilience.

5. Community and Peer Support:

- Mutual Support: Engaging with peer support groups or online communities of fellow cancer patients and survivors fosters mutual encouragement, shared experiences, and practical advice on coping strategies and resilience.

- Educational Resources: Accessing reliable information about cancer, treatment options, and self-care practices empowers individuals to make informed decisions and actively participate in their care, enhancing feelings of control and resilience.

By integrating these coping strategies and resilience-building techniques into their daily lives, individuals affected by cancer can cultivate inner strength, adaptability, and emotional well-being. These approaches complement medical treatment and support a holistic approach to cancer care that addresses the physical, emotional, and psychosocial needs of patients and survivors alike.

CHAPTER TEN

ADVANCES IN CANCER TREATMENT AND MANAGEMENT

overview of treatment options

1. Surgery:

=> Types of Surgical Interventions: Surgery is a cornerstone of cancer treatment, aiming to physically remove cancerous tissues from the body. It includes procedures such as:

- Primary Tumor Resection: Direct removal of the tumor and surrounding tissue, which is often curative in early-stage cancers localized to one area.

- Lymph Node Dissection: Removal of nearby lymph nodes to assess cancer spread and prevent further metastasis.

- Debulking Surgery: Reducing the size of tumors when complete removal isn't feasible, aiming to alleviate symptoms and improve response to other treatments like chemotherapy or radiation.

- Advancements in Surgical Techniques: Modern advancements like minimally invasive surgery (laparoscopy, robotic surgery) have revolutionized cancer surgery:

- Laparoscopic Surgery: Uses small incisions and a camera-guided scope to access tumors, reducing recovery time, pain, and risk of infection compared to traditional open surgery.

- Robotic Surgery: Provides surgeons with enhanced precision and control through robotic-assisted tools, allowing for complex procedures with minimal trauma to surrounding tissues.

- Role in Cancer Management: Surgery is

often the first-line treatment for solid tumors that are localized and operable. It may be curative in early-stage cancers or used as part of a multimodal approach alongside chemotherapy, radiation, or targeted therapies to achieve the best outcomes.

2. Chemotherapy:

=> Mechanism and Goals: Chemotherapy uses powerful drugs to kill fast-dividing cancer cells or inhibit their growth throughout the body:

- Systemic Treatment: Administered orally or intravenously, chemotherapy targets both primary tumors and metastatic cancer cells circulating in the bloodstream.

- Goals: Chemotherapy aims to shrink tumors before surgery (neoadjuvant therapy), eliminate residual cancer cells after surgery (adjuvant therapy), or control cancer growth and manage symptoms in advanced stages.

- Types of Chemotherapy Agents: Different classes of drugs target various aspects of cancer cell growth and replication:

- Alkylating Agents: Damage DNA to prevent cancer cells from reproducing.

- Antimetabolites: Interfere with DNA synthesis or repair, affecting cell division.

- Anthracyclines and Taxanes: Disrupt cellular processes essential for cancer cell survival and proliferation.

- Advancements: Advances in chemotherapy focus on improving drug delivery, minimizing side effects through targeted therapies (e.g., HER2-targeted therapies in breast cancer), and developing combination regimens tailored to specific cancer types and molecular profiles.

3. Radiation Therapy:

=> Principles of Radiation Therapy: Radiation therapy uses high-energy beams or particles to damage DNA within cancer cells:

- Local Treatment: Administered externally (external beam radiation therapy, EBRT) or internally (brachytherapy), radiation targets tumors while sparing surrounding healthy tissues.

- Mechanism: Radiation causes irreparable DNA damage in cancer cells, leading to cell death or reduced tumor size over time.

- Types of Radiation: Different techniques and modalities are used based on tumor size, location, and cancer type:

- Intensity-Modulated Radiation Therapy (IMRT): Delivers precise radiation doses to tumors with complex shapes or near critical organs, minimizing side effects.

- Stereotactic Body Radiation Therapy (SBRT): Uses highly focused radiation beams to treat small, localized tumors in fewer sessions, suitable for lung, liver, and spine tumors.

- Proton Therapy: Uses protons instead of traditional photons, delivering radiation more precisely and reducing exposure to healthy tissues, beneficial for pediatric cancers and tumors near critical organs.

- Advancements: Continuous advancements enhance radiation therapy's effectiveness and safety, including image-guided radiation therapy (IGRT) for real-time tumor tracking and adaptive radiation planning to adjust treatment based on tumor response and changes in anatomy.

4. Multimodal Approaches:

=>Combined Treatment Strategies: Many cancers require a combination of surgery, chemotherapy, and radiation therapy to achieve optimal outcomes:

- Neoadjuvant Therapy: Administered before surgery to shrink tumors, reduce surgical complications, and improve the chances of complete tumor removal.

- Adjuvant Therapy: Given after surgery to eradicate remaining cancer cells, lower the risk of recurrence, and enhance long-term survival.

- Sequential and Concurrent Therapies: Oncologists tailor treatment plans based on cancer stage, type, and patient health, aiming for maximum tumor control while minimizing treatment-related side effects.

- Personalized Medicine: Advances in molecular diagnostics (e.g., genetic testing, tumor profiling) allow for personalized treatment approaches that target specific genetic mutations or biomarkers driving cancer growth. This precision medicine approach enhances treatment efficacy and reduces unnecessary toxicity.

5. Emerging Trends and Personalized Medicine:

=> Precision Medicine: Tailors treatment plans to individual patients based on genetic, molecular, and cellular characteristics of their tumors:

- Genomic Profiling: Identifies specific genetic mutations or alterations that can be targeted with novel therapies, such as BRAF inhibitors in melanoma or EGFR inhibitors in lung cancer.

- Liquid Biopsies: Analyzes circulating tumor DNA or other biomarkers in blood to monitor treatment response, detect minimal residual disease, and guide therapeutic decisions.

- Immunotherapy and Targeted Therapies: Represents groundbreaking approaches in cancer treatment that harness the body's immune system or target specific pathways essential for cancer cell survival:

  - Immune Checkpoint Inhibitors: Block proteins that inhibit immune response, allowing T-cells to recognize and attack cancer cells more effectively.

  - CAR T-cell Therapy: Engineers a patient's T-cells to target and destroy cancer cells, particularly effective in hematologic malignancies like leukemia and lymphoma.

  - Monoclonal Antibodies: Attach to specific proteins on cancer cells, delivering cytotoxic agents or activating immune responses to eliminate tumors.

  - Clinical Trials and Innovation: Continual research and clinical trials evaluate novel therapies, combination treatments, and biomarkers predictive of treatment response, driving ongoing advancements in cancer care.

targeted therapies and immunotherapy

Targeted therapies are treatments that specifically target certain molecular pathways or genetic mutations that drive cancer growth. Unlike traditional chemotherapy, which affects all rapidly dividing cells (including healthy ones), targeted therapies aim to selectively interfere with cancer cell functions while minimizing damage to normal tissues. Here are some key categories and examples of targeted therapies:

1. Tyrosine Kinase Inhibitors (TKIs):

- Mechanism: TKIs block specific enzymes (tyrosine kinases) involved in signaling pathways that promote cancer cell growth and survival.

Examples:

~   Imatinib: Used in chronic myeloid leukemia (CML) by inhibiting the BCR-ABL fusion protein.

~ Erlotinib: Targets the EGFR pathway in non-small cell lung cancer (NSCLC).

~   Sunitinib: Inhibits multiple tyrosine kinases including VEGFR and PDGFR, used in renal cell carcinoma (RCC).

2. Monoclonal Antibodies:

- Mechanism: Monoclonal antibodies are designed to bind to specific proteins on cancer cells or immune cells, marking them for destruction or blocking their function.

Examples:

~   Trastuzumab: Targets HER2-positive breast cancer by blocking HER2 receptors.

~ Rituximab: Used in B-cell non-Hodgkin

lymphomas by targeting CD20 on B-cells.

~   Pembrolizumab: An immune checkpoint inhibitor that targets PD-1 in various cancers to enhance immune response.

3. Hormone Therapies:

-      Mechanism: Hormone therapies interfere with hormone production or block hormone receptors on cancer cells, which are crucial for hormone-sensitive cancers.

Examples:

~ Tamoxifen: Blocks estrogen receptors in estrogen receptor-positive breast cancers.

~   Enzalutamide: Inhibits androgen receptors in prostate cancer.

4. PARP Inhibitors:

- Mechanism: PARP inhibitors block an enzyme (poly ADP-ribose polymerase) involved in DNA repair, specifically in cancers with defects in DNA repair pathways like BRCA mutations.

Examples:

~ Olaparib: Used in ovarian and breast cancers with BRCA mutations.

~ Rucaparib: Also used in ovarian cancer with BRCA mutations.

Immunotherapy

Immunotherapy harnesses the body's immune system to recognize and attack cancer cells more effectively. These treatments aim to boost the immune response against tumors, overcome mechanisms that cancer cells use to evade detection, and induce long-lasting anti-cancer immunity. Here are the main types of immunotherapy:

1. Immune Checkpoint Inhibitors:

- Mechanism: Immune checkpoint inhibitors block inhibitory pathways (checkpoints) that dampen the immune response against cancer cells, allowing T-cells to remain active and attack tumors.

Examples:

~ Pembrolizumab: Targets PD-1/PD-L1 interactions in melanoma, NSCLC, and other cancers.

~ Nivolumab: Also targets PD-1 in melanoma, NSCLC, and others.

~ Ipilimumab: Targets CTLA-4 in melanoma and other cancers.

2. CAR T-cell Therapy:

- Mechanism: Chimeric Antigen Receptor (CAR) T-cell therapy involves genetically engineering a patient's T-cells to express receptors (CARs) that recognize specific proteins on cancer cells. Once infused back into the patient, CAR T-cells target and destroy cancer cells.

Examples:

~ Tisagenlecleucel (Kymriah): Approved for certain types of leukemia and lymphoma.

~ Axicabtagene ciloleucel (Yescarta): Approved for certain types of lymphoma.

3. Cytokine Therapy:

- Mechanism: Cytokines are proteins that regulate immune responses. Therapies involving cytokines aim to boost immune activity against cancer cells.

Examples

~ Interferons: Used in melanoma and

certain types of leukemia.

~   Interleukins: Used in renal cell carcinoma and melanoma.

4. Cancer Vaccines:

- Mechanism: Cancer vaccines aim to stimulate the immune system to recognize and attack cancer cells expressing specific antigens.

Examples:

~ Sipuleucel-T: Used in prostate cancer to stimulate an immune response against prostate-specific antigen (PSA).

~ GVAX: Investigational vaccines targeting specific tumor-associated antigens.

Advancements and Applications

- Personalized Medicine: Targeted therapies

and immunotherapies are central to the concept of personalized medicine, where treatment decisions are guided by genetic, molecular, and immune profiling of individual tumors.

- Combination Therapies: Many cancers benefit from combining targeted therapies with other treatments like chemotherapy, radiation, or other targeted agents to enhance efficacy and overcome resistance.

- Clinical Trials and Research: Ongoing research continues to identify new targets for therapy, improve treatment responses, and develop strategies to manage side effects and resistance mechanisms.

These therapies represent a paradigm shift in cancer treatment, offering more precise and effective options with potentially fewer side effects compared to traditional treatments. They highlight the importance of understanding the molecular and immune characteristics of tumors to tailor treatment strategies that maximize benefits for individual patients.

Integrative approaches to cancer care

These encompass a holistic and comprehensive approach that combines conventional medical treatments with complementary therapies and supportive care interventions. These approaches aim to address not only the physical aspects of cancer but also the emotional, psychological, and social needs of patients. Here's a detailed exploration of integrative approaches in cancer care:

Complementary Therapies

1. Mind-Body Practices:

- Meditation: Involves techniques to promote relaxation, reduce stress, and improve emotional well-being. Meditation may help patients cope with anxiety, depression, and treatment-related side effects.

- Yoga: Combines physical postures, breathing exercises, and meditation to enhance flexibility, strength, and overall quality of life. Yoga is also beneficial for managing fatigue, insomnia, and stress.

- Tai Chi: A mind-body practice that involves gentle movements, deep breathing, and meditation. Tai Chi improves balance, flexibility, and mental clarity while reducing stress levels.

2. Art Therapy and Creative Expression:

- Art Therapy: Utilizes creative processes

such as painting, drawing, and sculpting to facilitate emotional expression, reduce anxiety, and promote relaxation. Art therapy can help patients cope with trauma, grief, and existential concerns.

-   Music Therapy: Uses music interventions, including listening, playing instruments, or singing, to address emotional, physical, and social needs. Music therapy aids in pain management, stress reduction, and enhancing overall mood.

3. Nutritional Therapy:

-   Dietary Counseling: Provides personalized dietary recommendations to support overall health, optimize nutrition during treatment, and manage treatment-related side effects such as nausea, loss of appetite, and weight changes.

- Supplements: Certain vitamins, minerals, and herbal supplements may complement conventional treatments and support immune function. However, it's essential to consult healthcare providers to ensure safety and efficacy.

Supportive Care

1. Oncology Social Work:

   - Counseling and Support: Oncology social workers provide emotional support, counseling, and resources to help patients and families cope with the psychosocial challenges of cancer diagnosis, treatment, and survivorship.

   - Navigating Resources: They assist in navigating healthcare systems, accessing financial assistance programs, and connecting with community support services.

2. Pain Management:

- Palliative Care: Focuses on managing pain, symptoms, and improving quality of life for patients with advanced or terminal cancer. Palliative care integrates physical, emotional, and spiritual support to address holistic patient needs.

- Interventional Pain Management: Includes techniques such as nerve blocks, spinal cord stimulation, and medication adjustments to alleviate pain and improve comfort.

Traditional Medicine and Integrative Oncology

1. Traditional Chinese Medicine (TCM):

- Acupuncture: Involves inserting thin needles into specific points on the body to stimulate energy flow (Qi) and promote healing. Acupuncture may help manage pain, nausea, and fatigue in cancer patients.

- Herbal Medicine: Uses plant-based remedies to support immune function, reduce inflammation, and manage symptoms. Herbal formulations are tailored to individual patient needs and may be used in conjunction with conventional treatments.

2. Chiropractic Care and Physical Therapy:

- Chiropractic Care: Focuses on spinal alignment and musculoskeletal health. It can help alleviate pain, improve mobility, and enhance overall well-being during and after cancer treatment.

- Physical Therapy: Provides exercises, stretches, and manual techniques to improve strength, flexibility, and function. Physical therapy helps cancer survivors regain physical abilities and manage treatment-related impairments.

Psychosocial Support and Spiritual Care

1. Counseling and Psychotherapy:

   - Individual Therapy: Offers a confidential space for patients to explore feelings, cope with stress, and develop coping strategies. Cognitive-behavioral therapy (CBT) and other therapeutic approaches help patients adjust to cancer-related challenges.

   - Support Groups: Facilitate peer support, shared experiences, and coping strategies among individuals facing similar cancer diagnoses or treatment journeys.

2. Spiritual Care:

   - Pastoral Counseling: Provides spiritual guidance, comfort, and support to patients and families dealing with existential questions, grief, and end-of-life issues.

   - Mindfulness and Meditation: Cultivates present-moment awareness, acceptance, and spiritual connection. Spiritual practices can enhance resilience, inner peace, and overall well-being.

Research and Integration into Standard Care

Integrative approaches to cancer care are increasingly recognized and integrated into comprehensive cancer treatment plans. Research continues to explore the efficacy, safety, and potential benefits of these therapies in combination with conventional treatments. The goal is to provide personalized care that addresses the diverse needs of cancer patients, improves treatment outcomes, and enhances quality of life throughout the cancer journey.

CHAPTER ELEVEN

SURVIVORSHIP AND LONG-TERM CARE

Challenges faced by cancer survivors

Cancer survivors face a wide array of challenges that can significantly impact their quality of life and overall well-being. These challenges can be categorized into several key areas:

Physical Challenges

1. Long-Term Side Effects of Treatment: Many cancer treatments such as chemotherapy, radiation therapy, and surgery can cause persistent physical effects. These may include fatigue, pain, neuropathy, lymphedema (swelling), infertility, and cognitive difficulties (often

referred to as "chemo brain").

2. Increased Risk of Secondary Cancers: Some cancer survivors are at higher risk of developing secondary cancers due to treatment or genetic predispositions. Regular monitoring and preventive measures are essential.

3. Chronic Health Conditions: Treatment may predispose survivors to chronic conditions like cardiovascular disease, osteoporosis, and metabolic disorders.

Emotional and Psychological Challenges

1. Fear of Recurrence: The fear that cancer will return is a pervasive concern among survivors, impacting their emotional well-being and quality of life.

2. Anxiety and Depression: Coping with the trauma of cancer diagnosis and treatment can lead to anxiety disorders, depression,

post-traumatic stress disorder (PTSD), and adjustment disorders.

3. Body Image Issues: Physical changes due to treatment (e.g., scars, hair loss, weight changes, altered appearance) can affect self-esteem and body image.

Social and Practical Challenges

1. Financial Hardship: The cost of cancer treatment and ongoing medical care can lead to financial strain, especially if survivors experience reduced work capacity or job loss.

2. Changes in Relationships: Cancer can strain relationships with family, friends, and partners due to changes in roles, communication difficulties, and emotional stress.

3. Employment Issues: Survivors may face challenges in returning to work due to

physical limitations, cognitive impairment, or discrimination.

Survivorship and Long-Term Management

1. Access to Ongoing Care: Ensuring access to healthcare services for monitoring and managing long-term effects is crucial but may be challenging due to geographical, financial, or healthcare system barriers.

2. Health Promotion and Lifestyle Changes: Encouraging survivors to adopt healthy behaviors such as regular exercise, balanced nutrition, smoking cessation, and limiting alcohol intake to reduce the risk of recurrence and manage long-term health.

3. Navigating Survivorship Care Plans: Developing and implementing personalized survivorship care plans that address the survivor's medical history, treatment received, and potential long-term effects is essential for optimizing their health

outcomes.

In conclusion, addressing the multifaceted challenges faced by cancer survivors requires a comprehensive approach that integrates medical care, psychosocial support, and practical assistance. Supporting survivors through survivorship programs, rehabilitation services, counseling, and community resources can significantly enhance their overall well-being and quality of life post-cancer treatment.

Follow-up care and monitoring for cancer survivors

These are critical aspects of ensuring long-term health and detecting any potential recurrence or late effects of treatment. Here are more detailed aspects of follow-up care and monitoring:

1. **Frequency and Timing of Follow-Up Visits:**

- Follow-up schedules vary depending on the type of cancer, stage at diagnosis, and treatments received.

- Initially, follow-up visits may be frequent (e.g., every 3-6 months) and then become less frequent as time progresses and the risk of recurrence decreases.

2. **Components of Follow-Up Visits:**

- Physical Examination: Routine physical exams to check for any new symptoms or physical changes.

- Imaging Tests: Depending on the cancer type and stage, imaging such as CT scans, MRI, PET scans, or ultrasound may be performed periodically to detect any signs of recurrence.

- Laboratory Tests: Blood tests to monitor tumor markers or assess organ function, such as liver and kidney function tests.

3. **Monitoring for Late Effects of Treatment:**

- Cancer treatments such as chemotherapy, radiation therapy, and surgery can have long-term effects on various organs and systems.

- Monitoring may involve assessing cardiac function (especially after certain chemotherapies), bone health, cognitive function, and fertility issues.

4. **Psychosocial Support and Survivorship Care Planning:**

- Addressing emotional and psychological

needs through counseling, support groups, or referrals to mental health professionals.

   - Developing a survivorship care plan that outlines the individual's treatment history, potential late effects, and a plan for ongoing care and surveillance.

5. **Health Promotion and Lifestyle Counseling:**

   - Promoting healthy behaviors such as regular exercise, balanced nutrition, smoking cessation, and moderation in alcohol consumption to reduce the risk of recurrence and improve overall well-being.

   - Education on signs and symptoms of recurrence and when to seek medical attention promptly.

6. **Shared Care Model:**

- Collaboration between oncologists, primary care physicians, and other healthcare providers to ensure comprehensive and coordinated care.

- Transitioning from oncology-focused care to survivorship-focused care as the risk of recurrence decreases.

7. **Patient Education and Empowerment:**

- Empowering survivors with knowledge about their disease, treatment effects, and resources available for support.

- Encouraging self-management and adherence to recommended follow-up care guidelines.

Overall, follow-up care and monitoring aim to detect any recurrence early while managing and minimizing long-term effects of cancer treatment, thereby optimizing the survivor's quality of life and health outcomes in the long term.

Quality of life issues and survivorship programs

These are crucial aspects of cancer care that focus on enhancing well-being and supporting individuals post-treatment. Here's an exhaustive look at these topics:

Quality of Life Issues:

1. **Physical Well-being:**

- Symptom Management: Addressing pain, fatigue, nausea, and other physical symptoms resulting from cancer treatment.

- Rehabilitation: Physical therapy to regain strength, mobility, and function post-surgery or after prolonged treatment.

- Palliative Care: Providing relief from

symptoms and improving quality of life, focusing on comfort and dignity.

2. **Psychological and Emotional Health:**

- Psychosocial Support: Counseling, support groups, and therapies to manage anxiety, depression, fear of recurrence, and PTSD.

- Cognitive Function: Addressing "chemo brain" or cognitive impairments post-treatment through cognitive rehabilitation and strategies to improve memory and concentration.

3. **Social Well-being:**

- Support Systems: Building and maintaining relationships with family, friends, and support networks.

- Work and Financial Stability: Coping with changes in employment, financial strain due to medical bills, and navigating insurance coverage.

4. **Spiritual and Existential Concerns:**

- Existential Distress: Addressing issues related to meaning, purpose, and existential concerns arising from the cancer experience.

- Spiritual Care: Providing support for spiritual needs and beliefs, often through chaplaincy services or spiritual counselors.

5. **Sexual Health and Intimacy:**

- Sexual Dysfunction: Managing changes in libido, fertility, and physical intimacy due to cancer treatments.

- Education and Counseling: Providing

information and support for sexual health concerns, including body image issues.

6. **Nutritional Support:**

- Dietary Counseling: Promoting healthy eating habits tailored to individual needs and managing treatment-related side effects like taste changes or difficulty swallowing.

- Nutritional Supplements: Recommending supplements to address deficiencies and support overall health.

Survivorship Programs:

1. **Education and Information:**

- Providing survivors with comprehensive information about their diagnosis, treatment history, potential late effects, and long-term care plans.

- Empowering survivors to actively participate in their care and make informed decisions about lifestyle choices.

2. **Supportive Care:**

- Support Groups: Connecting survivors with peers who share similar experiences, providing emotional support and sharing coping strategies.

- Individual Counseling: Offering one-on-one sessions with psychologists or social workers to address specific concerns and mental health needs.

3. **Follow-Up Care and Monitoring:**

- Establishing regular follow-up visits to monitor for recurrence, manage late effects of treatment, and promote overall health.

- Coordination between oncologists, primary care providers, and other specialists to ensure comprehensive care.

4. **Rehabilitation Services:**

- Providing access to physical therapy, occupational therapy, and speech therapy to improve functional abilities and quality of life.

- Addressing rehabilitation needs specific to cancer treatments, such as lymphedema management or prosthetic services.

5. **Survivorship Care Plans:**

- Developing personalized survivorship care plans outlining individualized recommendations for ongoing care, surveillance, and health promotion.

- Including a summary of treatment received, potential late effects, and recommendations for follow-up care and healthy living.

6. **Health Promotion and Wellness Activities:**

- Encouraging survivors to engage in healthy behaviors such as regular exercise, balanced nutrition, smoking cessation, and stress management.

- Offering wellness programs, workshops, or seminars on topics relevant to survivorship, such as mindfulness, yoga, or relaxation techniques.

7. **Advocacy and Resources:**

- Advocating for survivors' needs within healthcare systems and communities to ensure access to supportive services, financial assistance, and survivorship resources.

- Connecting survivors with community organizations, online resources, and national support networks for additional information and support.

In conclusion, quality of life issues and survivorship programs play integral roles in supporting cancer survivors beyond their initial treatment phase, aiming to enhance overall well-being, manage treatment-related effects, and promote a fulfilling life post-cancer. These programs underscore the importance of holistic care and personalized support to optimize survivor outcomes and quality of life.

REFERENCES

Michael B. Sporn and Anita B. Roberts (2003). Chemoprevention of Cancer: A

Clinical Update.

Michael T. Lotze and Augustine M.K. Choi (2007). Cancer Immunosurveillance and

Immunoediting: Therapeutic

Implications.

David S. Alberts, Lisa M. Hess, and Susan J. Ramondetta (2017). Gynecologic

Oncology: Clinical Practice and

Surgical Atlas.

Robert G. Bristow, Anil K. Sood, and David M. Gershenson (2019). Diagnosis and

Management of Ovarian

Disorders.

Elizabeth A. Platz, Meir J. Stampfer, and Walter C. Willett (2020). Epidemiology of

Cancer.

Vincent T. DeVita Jr., Theodore S. Lawrence, and Steven A. Rosenberg (2020). DeVita, Hellman, and Rosenberg's

Cancer: Principles & Practice

of Oncology.

Sidney Farber, Robert A. Weinberg, and Ronald A. DePinho (2015). The Molecular

Basis of Cancer.

Douglas R. Lowy, John T. Schiller (2006).

HPV Vaccines: Issues and

Perspectives"

Margaret L. Kripke, Scott M. Lippman, and Ernest T. Hawk (2017). Cancer Prevention:

The Causes and Prevention of Cancer.

Ahmedin Jemal, Freddie Bray, Melissa M. Center, Jacques Ferlay, Elizabeth Ward, and David Forman (2021). Global Cancer Statistics 2020: GLOBOCAN Estimates of Incidence and Mortality Worldwide for 36 Cancers in 185 Countries.

Julie A. Ross, Peter D. Inskip, and Mark P. Little (2017). Cancer Epidemiology and Prevention

Bernard W. Stewart and Christopher P. Wild (2020). World Cancer Report.

Jean L. Bolognia, Julie V. Schaffer, and Lorenzo Cerroni (2018). Dermatology.

Michael J. Thun, Martha S. Linet, James R. Cerhan, and Christopher A. Haiman (2017).

Cancer Epidemiology and

Prevention.

Josep M. Llovet and Jordi Bruix (2019).

Hepatocellular Carcinoma:

Diagnosis and Treatment

Daniel G. Haller, Giuseppe Giaccone, and
Michael A. Choti (2006). Textbook of

Uncommon Cancer.

David Khayat, Salvatore T. Scagliotti, and
Heine H. Hansen (2019). Cancer

Prevention and Management

through Exercise and Weight

Control.

Brian Kavanagh, Kie Kian Ang, and Quynh-
Thu Le (2020). Principles and Practice of

Radiation Oncology.

Steven D. Shapiro, Judith D. Salerno, and

Louis J. DeGennaro (2019). Cancer

Prevention and Management

through Diet and Lifestyle.